Ketogenic Diet:
Beginner's Guide with 30 Recipes
Includes 10 Bonus Recipes

Disclaimer and Terms of Use:

Effort has been made to ensure that the information in this book is accurate and complete, however, the author and the publisher do not warrant the accuracy of the information, text and graphics contained within the book due to the rapidly changing nature of science, research, known and unknown facts and internet. The Author and the publisher do not hold any responsibility for errors, omissions or contrary interpretation of the subject matter herein. This book is presented solely for motivational and informational purposes only.

TABLE OF CONTENTS

Introduction

Ketogenic diet is a type of dieting program developed to promote the state of "ketosis", which aids in weight loss by making the body burn body fats rather than carbohydrates. This diet has created a breakthrough due to its proven effectiveness. However, it must be noted that the rate of weight loss depends on several factors, such as your metabolism rate and the amount of fat you want to get rid of.

In this diet, you are allowed to consume a low carbohydrate diet, moderate protein and high-fat diet in order to put your body into ketosis. Most people refer to it as the low-carb diet due to its nature.

By eating fewer carbs, the ketone levels in the body are heightened. Anyone who is in the ketogenic diet needs to achieve ketosis for the diet to take effect.

Basically, the ketogenic works only if the body gets into the state of ketosis. How does this take place?

Well, the body depends on glucose as its main fuel - glucose is produced by the break-down of carbohydrates and transformed into energy, which the body uses to power the organs and muscles. When the intake of carbs is limited, there will be a shortage in glucose. When this happens, the liver will produce ketones, which make the body burn fats for fuel instead. Thus, there can be a quick reduction in weight and body fats.

It must be noted that ketones are acidic compounds and may lead to serious problems. If ketone levels are neglected, you may suffer from heightened blood acidity and other problems related to kidney and the liver. Yet, when used properly and with full responsibility, this diet can have tons of beneficial effects to health, not only in losing weight.

In fact, it does not only help in dealing with conditions light excessive weight and obesity as well as epilepsy. The diet has also been found to have good effects in cardiovascular diseases as well as type 2 diabetes.

On an average, the body can attain desirable ketone levels for weight loss and other conditions within a period of 2-4 weeks. Any person on a ketogenic diet should maintain a certain ketone level, which is at 0.5 to 3mmol/L. But then, some people experience no problems having ketone levels at 5mmol/L.

Measuring the amount of ketones in your body is very easy. You may use a urine dipstick kit, which is both affordable and reliable method. There are also the blood test kits, but these are a bit more expensive.

How the Ketogenic Diet Works

The ketogenic diet program is very simple - low carbohydrate diet, which allows you to consume real food. If you are the type of person who has been used to eating a diet rich in carbohydrates, or perhaps you are one of those fat phobic dieters out there, well you will really benefit a lot from this section.

In the ketogenic diet, you need to be a bit more specific about the amount of carbs, proteins and fats that you eat as well as your caloric intake. So, before anything else, take a look at these:

a) Carbohydrates: A gram of carbohydrate is equivalent to 4 calories
b) Proteins: A gram of protein is equivalent to 4 calories
c) Fats: A gram of fat is equivalent to 9 calories

Now, the question is how much you should consume? Well, basically, simply stick to 10% calories coming from carbs, 30% from protein and 60% from fats. However, you should not rush things as your body may not be able to compensate for the change. The best thing that you can do is to trim down your carb intake by 50% and then go lower after a few days until you reach the target limit that helps your body maintain ketosis. If your allowable carb intake is so low, make sure you avoid too many fruits and carb loaded treats.

Stay moderate on your protein intake - ideally you should consume 1 to 2 grams of protein per 1 kilogram of body weight. If you weigh 50 kg, you should be eating about 50 to 100 grams of protein.

While, 60% of your diet should be composed of fats - don't feel bad with this because you need lots of fats to keep your body in ketosis. After all, these fats get burned during the process. However, you should consume healthy fats, like omega 3s saturated and monounsaturated ones.

Unlike other diets, you do not have to control the amount of food that you eat in a deliberate manner. But then, you should know when to stop when your tummy is already full, even when there is still food on your plate. The simplest rule is: just eat when you feel hungry and never let other people influence you on how frequent or what you eat.

Also, there is no need to strictly count your calorie intake while trying to lose weight using this diet. But you need to watch on calories when you already achieved your weight goal. Of course, your body needs to adjust according to its needs.

Another thing that you should remember is to drink lots of water - as much as possible drink 2 to 3 liters per day.

You can't simply jump into the ketogenic diet without knowing about the essentials. This low carb diet thing is very simple, yet there are still measures that you need to observe. Before you begin dieting, here are a few things that you should bear in mind:

Take care of your electrolytes

The three macronutrients, such as carbs, proteins and fat are not the only areas that you should look into as vitamins, minerals as well as electrolytes in the body are important as well.

Electrolytes, such as potassium, sodium and magnesium are often excreted excessively when under the ketogenic diet - particularly if you are consuming less than 20g of carbohydrates.

To replenish the potassium in your body, you may take cantaloupes, mushroom and avocado and fish, like salmon. Or, simply mix a pinch of salt in a liter of water - the same thing to do with sodium deficiency. If you lack magnesium, consume a handful of nuts each day or take magnesium supplements. Make sure you do not exceed the recommended daily allowance!

Don't rely too much on low-carb products

Make it a habit to stick to unprocessed food and be aware of deceptive labeling. There are a lot of products labeled as "low carbs", but this is not just true. More often than that, these products have higher carb content than stated in the label. Also, stay away from aspartame and other artificial additives and flavorings as these can have detrimental effects not only on your body weight, but your overall health as well.

Basically, you should avoid anything that is low carb or fat-free as these food items usually have additives and not satiating at all making you hungry more often, so your cravings can be triggered too.

Always plan ahead

You should make an effort to plan in advance to help you get a good start with the ketogenic diet. The first step that you may take is to eliminate everything that is not allowed in the diet, such as sugary foods, sugar, flour and processed foods among others. In short, get rid of anything that is tempting.

To avoid temptations, you should a plan or a list of foods to buy and meals to prepare for the whole week ahead. Don't go food shopping without something planned in mind as this will lead you to buying and eating foods that are not suitable for the ketogenic diet.

Carbs

There are many recommendations on how much you need to limit your carbohydrates in order to reach ketosis. Some suggest that all you need to do is lower your carbohydrate intake to less than 50 grams, some will even tell you that 100 grams or less is fine.

But the truth is that no one knows for sure because it varies from person to person. No one person is the same. We all have different levels of carbohydrate tolerance. The vast majority will need to keep their carbs under 50 grams, usually around 30 grams, but ultimately you will have to determine this for yourself by testing.

Your best bet is to start at about 40 grams of total carbs daily and adjust from there. After two weeks, if you are not producing enough ketones (below you'll learn how to measure them), slowly reduce your carbs by 5 grams a week until you do.

Protein intake

Despite what you may have heard, the ketogenic diet is NOT a high protein diet. In fact, eating too much protein can be a problem for some people, especially for those who are already sensitive to carbohydrates.

The problem with proteins is that your body, being the incredibly efficient machine that it is, has the ability to turn proteins into glucose (known as gluconeogenesis). Too much glucose can raise your insulin levels, preventing your body's ability to release and burn the fatty acids which leads to ketosis.

The amount of protein that causes gluconeogenesis varies from person to person, and depends on how insulin resistant you are.

To be safe, keep your protein consumption moderate at about .80 to 1.0 grams per each pound of lean body weight (depending on your activity level). If you work out and lift weights 3 times a week, use the higher number.

For example, if your lean body mass is 150 lbs.:

150 lbs. x .80 grams of protein =120 grams of protein per day or

150 lbs. x 1.0 grams protein =150 grams of protein per day

Calorie counting

Some will argue that calorie counting is not really necessary on a ketogenic diet, but if your goal is to lose weight then the law of thermogenics still applies.

Although many people report that they have successfully lost weight without counting calories, it's probably due to the fact that people did not eat as much because the ketogenic diet is very satisfying. And also because they did not have to deal with the constant insulin spikes caused by carbohydrates, they were not as hungry and tempted to cheat. Ketones also dampen your appetite.

However, we still recommend you start out with a moderate calorie deficit. Severely cutting back your calories is never a good idea and will usually backfire on you in the long run, causing metabolic damage.

Start with a calorie deficit of no more than 15-20% below maintenance levels. You can get a close approximation of your maintenance calories by multiplying your current weight by 15 or 16. Then multiply that number by .80 (80%) to give you a 20% deficit.

Example using the values for maintenance calories from the last section:

Female at 150 lbs. x 15 cal/lb. = 2250 cal/day.

A 20% deficit is 2250 x 0.80 = 1800

1800 calories/day

Male at 180 lbs. x 16 cal/lb. = 2880 cal/day

A 15% deficit is 2880 cal/day x 0.85 = 2448

2448 calories/day

These figures should be considered starting points only as they are based on averages and estimations for maintenance calorie levels. Some individuals may need to reduce calories further.

How are ketones measured?

Ketones are only produced when the insulin levels are low. A sure sign of low insulin is a high amount of ketones in the bloodstream. When your ketones are high, it is referred to as optimal ketosis.

So how do you know whether or not you have a healthy amount of ketones in your bloodstream? The traditional way of checking is through a urine sample using urine test sticks (ketosis). They are the easiest to start with and you can buy them at any drugstore.

However, the longer you stay in ketosis, the less reliable urine sticks become because the kidneys become more efficient at absorbing ketones and fewer will show up in your urine. You may end up mistakenly thinking that ketosis is slowing when in fact your body has just adapted to using ketones as its main energy source.

If you want a more accurate measure, there are many test gadgets that will test your blood for ketones that are now available for home use. They are reasonably priced as well. All it takes is a prick of your finger.

It is ideal to measure your blood ketones in the morning on an empty stomach. If your blood ketone test result is at 1.5 to 3.0mmol/L, you are in an optimal ketosis, which means your body has reached a level ideal for maximum weight loss.

This is what you should be aiming for if you want to stop stalling and get over a weight loss plateau. Anything below or above these values is not recommended. That would mean you are still either getting a little more carbs or not getting an adequate amount of food.

For instance, blood ketones of 0.5mmol/L or below are not a ketosis level. At this point, you are not losing or burning fat. If your blood ketone is between 0.5 and 1.5mmol/L, you may be losing weight but you can do better. This is considered a light nutritional ketosis. It is ideal for fat burning but not an optimal one.

On the other hand, if your blood ketone level is above 3.0mmol/L then you've officially gone overboard and it's no longer healthy.

Additional reminders

a) The list of things to observe when under the ketogenic diet is almost endless. To further guide you as you start on this dieting program, take a look at these:
b) Eat meat, eggs and vegetables without much starch - these are good for you!
c) Snack on nuts, like almonds and macadamia as well as fruits, like avocados.
d) Don't be fat phobic! Use lard, coconut oil and palm oil with your cooking.
e) When eating salad, grab some sesame oil, olive oil or anything organic.
f) Avoid trans-fats as well as processed oils like margarine and hydrogenated oil.

What about Weight Loss?

If you're interested in losing weight, then you no doubt know the magic number for weight loss: to lose a pound of mass, you have to burn 3,500 more calories than you take in.

However, if you look around, not everyone appears to be carrying their weight the same way. Some of this comes from genetics, and some of this comes from lifestyle choices. Some people have a body type that amasses fat in the belly area, while others take fat on more uniformly across their bodies.

While you can't fight your genes, you can make the right lifestyle choices when it comes to the fat that you take in, and starting a ketogenic diet is one of the best choices you can make when it comes to removing your belly fat quickly. It is important to realize that hormones tell our body what to do with the food that comes in.

One of the most important hormones in this area is insulin. When you take in glucose, your body releases insulin, and any carbohydrates that you consume break down into glucose. The more glucose you have in your bloodstream, the more insulin your body sets loose. Your body has to deal with glucose, because if the levels get too high, glucose becomes a toxin.

As a result, your liver and muscles can store it, or your body can burn it through metabolic processes, or you can store it as fat. Because you're converting your body to ketosis, though, you won't burn glucose - but fat instead. You're going to bring your carb consumption down close to zero, which means that the insulin hormone won't be circulating through your blood telling your body to shove fat into a place you don't want it. Instead, you'll be burning it.

This is why the ketogenic diet is one of the best ways to shed belly fat. Any low carb diet limits the glucose you're taking in, keeping you from spiking in glucose (and then spiking in insulin, and then storing glucose as fat).

A recent discovery of how insulin works makes it simple to understand why so many people in the West have issues with weight. So many meals have more than 100 grams of carbohydrates that digest quickly and then absorb as fat.

Pizza, sandwich bread, hamburger buns, noodles, cereals, and drinks with sugar all tell your body to send insulin around the body. These foods all contain processed carbohydrates. Because the body has an easier time breaking these down, the glucose inside hits our bloodstream more quickly and in greater volume than fruits and vegetables - even the starchy and sugary ones.

If you drink a 20 ounce bottle of Coke or Sprite, you are taking in as much sugar as you would by eating nine cups of strawberries. Remember that glucose is ultimately toxic if the levels get to high, so your body has to figure out what to do with it. When you exercise, you use the glucose that is in your muscles and then liver. If those areas have little or no glucose left, what you take in goes to those repositories before it goes to fat.

The average active person only needs 150 grams of carbohydrates each day to keep full levels of glycogen in the liver and muscles. In the West, the average person takes in about 300 grams of carbohydrates on a daily basis. Their activity levels are low (no, Facebooking doesn't count as exercise). This means that each meal adds more glucose into your fat storage area. Also, every meal is followed by the introduction of a hormone (insulin) that hinders you from burning fat as energy. Wonder why it's so hard to lose weight?

You may also have read about the increasing number of cases of type 2 diabetes among Western societies. This increase is a direct consequence of the ways our diet influences our insulin. If you have habitually eaten a high carb diet, you have likely built up some degree of insulin resistance. You feel lethargic, gain weight and are at risk of type 2 diabetes. The good news is that this is easy to turn around with a ketogenic diet.

Another hormone that is important to understand when you are thinking about burning belly fat is Cortisol. This is the hormone that your body uses to signal the need to release the energy that is being stored inside fat cells. Your Cortisol levels are highest first thing in the morning, but any time your body has stress that is physical or mental, Cortisol enters the system as well. Balanced Cortisol levels are a good thing.

However, because of the high levels of stress that are a part of modern life for too many of us, it is easy for Cortisol levels to get out of control.

When your Cortisol levels are too high, your body will fight fat loss, and you will gain more weight. If there is a layer of fat on your belly that you just cannot lose, no matter how hard you exercise or how well you diet, your Cortisol levels are probably too high.

So how does the ketogenic diet interact with these hormones? The magic word here is leptin. This is the hormone that tells you to stop eating because you are full. Your body sends out a lot of leptin when you take in proteins and fats and a little when you take in carbohydrates.

Think about it. Would you be able to eat more slices of bacon or French toast sticks? Which would make you feel full (or even a little green at the gills) faster? The bacon will make you feel full sooner, and you'll feel full longer.

This is why so many healthy snacks for weight loss have protein in them, because they signal your body to send out leptin so you don't go back to the pantry for chips after you have your snack. Staying away from carbs and sticking with high protein and high fat meals, you stop eating sooner, your blood glucose levels stay manageable, and that belly fat starts to fall away, particularly if you stick with a regular exercise regimen.

Getting Started

Congratulations! You should now have a pretty good understanding of how the ketogenic diet works and be ready to get started. The following tips will help you get prepared for success.

Clear out the kitchen

If you have tried a low carb diet before then you are already familiar with the drill. In a ketogenic diet, carb consumption is ideally around 30-40 grams and almost always below 50. Start by clearing your kitchen of any high carb foods. Again, complex carbohydrates are not allowed so steer clear of them. Put them away for now.

Next, you have to start restocking your kitchen with low carb foods. Stick with vegetables as much as possible. And don't forget about your protein and fat sources too. You don't necessarily have to spend a ton of money on special foods. But when you do your grocery shopping, stick with artificial ingredient-free foods. Choose real foods and forget anything says it's "low carb". As a rule, if it's marked low carb on the package, you shouldn't be eating it.

In order to keep track of your carb intake, it is recommended that you get yourself a carb counter guide. This will help you monitor your carb consumption with every food or meal you take so you can stay within the limits.

Plan your meals ahead

If you only spend time in the kitchen when eating, you have to change that now. This diet requires you to spend a little more time in this area of the house. You are encouraged to cook your own meals. That is the best way to keep count of your carb, fat and protein intake.

It is important that you plan your meals ahead of time.

Keep these rules in mind when planning your meals: 60-65 percent of caloric consumption must come from fat, 30 percent should be obtained from protein and the remaining 5-10 percent should consist of carbohydrates.

Drink plenty of water

Since your carb consumption will be reduced, there is a tendency that your kidneys will eliminate excess water it may have held up when you were still eating an unlimited amount of carbs. In which case, it is recommended that you hydrate properly. It is important that you replace the fluids your body loses in the process.

Do not wait until you feel the thirst. Make it a point to drink at least eight glasses of water a day. When you experience muscle cramps and headaches, you are likely losing water. And when you do drink water, you are also advised to take minerals including potassium, magnesium and salt. That's because these minerals get swept away along with water.

Now if you are not too keen about drinking tasteless water, you can always increase your fluid intake through green juices and smoothies. Get juice from high water vegetables such as cucumbers. And you can make smoothies out of any available ingredients around your kitchen. It is also a good way of increasing your vegetable intake.

Don't exercise for the first 2 weeks

This diet puts your body through a lot of changes. You have to give it time to adjust. Do not push yourself to exercise for the first few weeks into the diet. Otherwise, you are only causing unnecessary stress.

Other tips

As mentioned, you are discouraged from exercising at least for the first few weeks into the diet. The first 2 to 3 weeks are crucial because your body goes through what is called a metabolic shift. And during this phase, you should expect to experience brain fog and fatigue.

Watch out for other side effects which may include dizziness, general lethargy and flu-like symptoms. Most of the time, these are signs of dehydration. To increase water retention, you may want to salt everything starting with the water you drink. As your body gets used to the diet and all the changes it brings, these side effects should go away.

Also, because of the limit in carb intake, your body may experience a micronutrient deficiency. And this is why you are encouraged to supplement. Choose a high quality multivitamin with minerals and make sure your body is getting enough fiber by eating plenty of fiber rich green vegetables.

Finally, do not let your blood ketone get out of control. Monitor it regularly. If you go beyond the optimal ketosis level, you are at risk to ketoacidosis.

Recipes

Breakfast

Breakfast is the most important meal of the day and this principle also applies with the ketogenic diet. Whether you are in a hurry or have a little time to spare for breakfast, you will absolutely enjoy the following recipes. You will surely find one that matches the kind of morning you are having.

Sausage patties

Free from gluten and soy content, this breakfast sausage is perfectly fit for someone trying to lose weight. It is easy and you can make it ahead of time *and* store in the refrigerator. This recipe yields 15 servings.

Ingredients:

2 pounds of ground chicken sausage

1/4 cup of white finely chopped onion

3 garlic cloves, finely minced

1 tablespoon of ground sage

1/2 tablespoon of finely minced rosemary

1 tablespoon salt

1/2 tablespoon freshly ground black pepper

Put all the ingredients in a large bowl. Mix well until the seasonings are well combined with the meat. Divide the mixture into 7 equal portions. You can use an ice cream scoop for this process. Press on the mixture to form a patty.

Arrange the patties on a waxed cookie sheet. Store the patties by stacking them together, separating one from the other by placing a paper after each patty layer. Then, cover the entire stack using a plastic wrap. Place in the fridge for at least 2 hours.

You can cook these sausage patties immediately after taking them out of the fridge. Use a lidded pan for cooking over medium heat. Each side of the patty must be cooked for 6 or 7 minutes.

Breakfast casserole

The usual casserole recipes are filled with cheese, making them fattening. This casserole recipe is not only a much healthier alternative, it is also very delicious. The only downside is it takes some time to prepare and cook. You need to spare a total of 55 minutes for both prep and cooking. This recipe yields 2 servings.

Ingredients:

5 eggs

3 bacon strips, cooked

1 cup fresh baby spinach

1/2 cup butternut squash, chopped

1/2 cup fresh mushrooms, sliced

1/2 cup yellow squash, chopped

1/4 cup red onion, chopped

1 pinch garlic powder

Salt and pepper to taste

Pre-heat the oven first to 350 degrees. Combine all the ingredients in a medium sized bowl except for the seasoning. Mix well. Next, add garlic powder with salt and pepper to taste.

Brush the bottom and sides of the baking dish with coconut oil. Pour the mixture. Put inside the pre-heated oven. Let it cook at 350 degrees for 45 minutes. When cooked, place in a cooling rack, then serve.

Chia breakfast

This breakfast recipe is ideal for busy mornings. If you're used to oatmeal, this is your healthier option. It's so easy to prepare, it will only take ten minutes or less of your time. This recipe is good for two.

Ingredients:

1 cup boiling water

1/2 cup almond milk, unsweetened

4 tablespoons of Chia seeds

4 tablespoons shredded coconut, unsweetened

4 tablespoons flax meal

1 tablespoon cinnamon

Stevia

Mix all the ingredients in a bowl except for the water and almond milk. Make sure the mixture is well blended. Now pour the boiling water into the mixture. Stir it well. Set it aside for 3 minutes then stir.

Add the almond milk then stir and serve.

Spinach and mushroom quiche

This is another easy breakfast recipe you can make in 40 minutes. This recipe serves two.

Ingredients:

    6 large eggs

    3 white mushrooms, sliced

    1/2 medium onion, finely chopped

    1 cup of chopped fresh spinach

    1/2 cup unsweetened almond milk

    1/2 teaspoon baking powder

    Salt and pepper

Preheat the oven to 350 degrees Fahrenheit. Beat the eggs in a bowl then add the coconut milk. Whisk together using a hand mixer. Add the rest of the ingredients one by one as you continue stirring.

Apply grease on a baking dish. Pour the quiche mixture into the baking dish then bake for about 40 minutes. You can take this breakfast dish to go by slicing the quiche into squares before storing them in a Ziploc bag.

Low carb breakfast bar

This is one of the most convenient breakfast recipes in the list. You can make this breakfast in less than 20 minutes. This recipe yields 5 servings.

Ingredients:

1 large egg

1/4 creamy roasted almond butter

1/2 tablespoon cinnamon

1/2 teaspoon vanilla

1/4 teaspoon baking soda

Sea salt

Stevia

Put the almond butter in a medium sized bowl and blend until creamy. Add egg, vanilla, honey and stevia then stir. You can also use a blender to make sure the ingredients are well blended. Then, add grease to a baking dish. Pour the batter into the dish and put in the oven. Let it cook at 325 degrees Fahrenheit for 12 to 15 minutes. Place in a cooling rack then divide into 5 equal portions. Enjoy!

Cucumber and strawberry salad

This breakfast is perfect for a lazy Sunday morning. It is especially good when the weather is hot. This refreshing salad is ideal as a light breakfast or side dish to a grilled food. This recipe serves two.

Ingredients:

1/2 cucumber, peeled and sliced

2 fresh strawberries, sliced

1/2 green bell pepper, diced

2 tablespoons freshly squeezed lime juice

Sesame seeds

Put the green bell pepper in a small bowl and drizzle with lime juice. Mix well. Combine the strawberries and cucumber in the bowl and mix. Then, add the pepper and lime mixture.

Toss until ingredients are well coated. Let it chill in the fridge for a few minutes. Sprinkle with sesame seeds before serving. If you like your breakfast with a creamy flavor, feel free to add feta cheese.

Winter sunshine smoothie

Ingredients:

2 peeled oranges

meat of a young Thai coconut

2 peeled bananas, you can also use frozen banana instead of ice cubes

A cup of ice

A cup of reserved coconut water, add more if needed

2 tablespoons of goji berries

1/4 cup of hemp seeds

1/4 cup beet kvass

1/4 teaspoon of turmeric

Put all the ingredients in the blender and blend until smooth and creamy. Add in the beet kvass and continue blending.

Sausage maple muffins

Ingredients:

- 6 ounces of ground sausage
- 4 tablespoons of coconut milk
- 4 eggs, large-sized
- 2 tablespoons of psyllium husk powder
- 4 tablespoons of maple syrup
- 1 teaspoon of baking powder
- 1 teaspoon of vanilla extract
- 1 and 1/2 cups of almond flour
- 1 /4 cup of erythritol
- 20 drops stevia (liquid)
- 1/4 teaspoon of salt

Break the sausages into small pieces.

Fry the outsides of the sausage in a hot pan and make sure you cook until crisp but not cook the inside completely.

Preheat your oven to 350F.

Prepare your 4 tablespoons of maple syrup, 4 eggs, 4 tablespoons of coconut milk, 20 drops liquid stevia, and 1 teaspoon of vanilla extract. Mix well until fully combined.

Prepare the dry ingredients: erythritol, almond flour, psyllium husk powder, and the baking powder.

Mix the dry and wet ingredients. Mix in the cooked sausages.

Put the mixtures into 12 silicone cupcake molds and put them in the oven to bake for around 20 to 25 minutes.

Let it cool for a few minutes after baking and remove from the molds. Serve and enjoy with a dash of maple syrup.

The Ketogenic Coffee

Ingredients:

A cup of coffee that is freshly brewed, (8 to 12 oz)

A tablespoon of butter, unsalted

A tablespoon of coconut oil, MCT

Put the MCT oil and butter with the coffee in the blender and blend until creamy and make sure there is no oil sitting on its surface. This takes around 20 seconds.

Serve immediately.

Breakfast bread

Ingredients:

Half cup of roasted almond butter

1/4 tsp. of sea salt

2 pieces of large eggs

1/4 tsp. of stevia

2 tbsp. of honey

1/4 tsp. of baking soda

A tsp. of vanilla extract

A tbsp. of ground cinnamon

Instructions:

Pour in the almond butter in a big bowl and mix until creamy.

Add in the honey, eggs, stevia, and vanilla.

Put the cinnamon, baking soda and salt.

Combine well with the hand blender until the ingredients are fully mixed.

Put the batter in a greased 8x8" baking dish. Bake for 12-15 minutes at 325 degrees.

Serve and enjoy.

Lunch

You need time to plan your lunch ahead. When you prepare in advance, you can choose healthier options as well as save money. Make sure you have healthy ingredients on hand.

Make sure your lunch is packed with protein to help fill you up. Protein also makes you feel satisfied for a longer period of time. Choose lean protein sources. Use a variety of fruits and vegetables as ingredients too. That said, below is a list of lunch recipes that are both nutritious and delicious.

Bulgarian ground meat

This recipe adds a whole new meaning to dieting. The mix of herbs and spices lends an interesting flavor to the meat. Add a fresh side salad to this and it is one you will love.

Ingredients:

- 1/4 pound ground beef

- 1 egg

- 1/2 onion, chopped

- 1/4 tablespoon dried thyme

- Ginger, coriander and ground cumin

- Salt and pepper to taste

Combine the ingredients in a large bowl. If you feel the mixture requires additional eggs, feel free to add. Scoop the mixture into the bread slices. Put it in the oven and bake the sandwich at medium heat for 7 minutes or until the meat is cooked through. Serve and enjoy!

Crab cakes

The key to successful dieting is variety. Here's a sumptuous crab cake recipe you will surely enjoy.

Ingredients:

   1/2 pound crab meat

   1 medium egg

   1/8 cup breadcrumbs (made from almond flour)

   1 tablespoon olive oil

   1 tablespoon mayonnaise

   1/2 tablespoon diced celery

   1/2 tablespoon minced onion

   1/4 tablespoon minced garlic

   1/2 teaspoon Old Bay Seasoning

   1/2 teaspoon Dijon mustard

   Salt and pepper

Combine the ingredients in a large bowl without the breadcrumbs and crab meat. Mix well then add crab meat. Mix again then gradually add the breadcrumbs.

Scoop the mixture into equal portions. Shape each portion into a ball and flatten to form cakes with half inch thickness.

Heat the pan and add olive oil. When the oil is hot enough, cook the crab cakes until each side is golden brown. Cook two cakes at a time. Serve immediately!

Thai style shrimp salad

If you are craving a little spice, you will absolutely love this Thai recipe. A well balanced flavor with just the right amount of spice, this salad is surely satisfying. This recipe is good for two.

Ingredients:

   1/2 pound steamed shrimp, cleaned and deveined

   1/2 head lettuce, cut into small pieces

   1/2 stalk lemongrass, sliced

1 red onion, sliced

1/4 inch ginger root, cut into small pieces

1 fresh red chili, sliced

1 garlic clove, crushed and minced

7 mint leaves

1 and 1/2 teaspoon lime juice

2 tablespoons chopped green onions

2 tablespoons chopped fresh cilantro

1 tablespoon fish sauce

Black pepper

Lay the lettuce leaves flat and arrange the shrimp over it. Pour the ginger, chili and onion on top. Set aside.

In the meantime, prepare the dressing. Combine the lime juice, lemongrass, garlic, pepper, and fish sauce together in a bowl. Mix well then pour over the shrimp salad. Add the cilantro, onion and mint leaves to garnish and serve.

Mexican ceviche

This seafood dish is commonly served on the beaches of Mexico. It is best served with sweet potato, lettuce or avocado and other side dishes that can complement its interesting flavors. If you want something different from your usual lunch, you have to give this dish a shot. And when you do, make sure you only use the freshest ingredients. This recipe is good for one.

Ingredients:

1/4 pound halibut fillet

1 lime

1 jalapeno pepper, finely chopped

1/2 small onion, finely chopped

1/4 green bell pepper, finely chopped

1/4 cup fresh tomato, finely sliced

1 tablespoon chopped parsley

1/2 chopped fresh cilantro

1/2 tablespoon white vinegar

1/8 teaspoon oregano

Salt and pepper

Lettuce leaf

Avocado and black olives for garnishing

Cut the fish into pieces. Each piece should be about half an inch. Squeeze lime juice over the fish. Stir. Then, store in the fridge overnight.

Before lunchtime, take the fish out and drain. Add the rest of the ingredients except for the avocado, lettuce and olives. Toss well. Arrange the lettuce on a serving dish. Lay it flat and pour the fish mixture over it. Add the black olives and avocado slices for garnishing. Serve and enjoy!

Black bean garlic sauce with Brussels sprouts

The flavor of the black bean garlic sauce goes perfectly well with the sprouts. There is no need to add salt because the sauce itself adds just enough flavor. If you want to try a little taste of Asian food, this recipe is a good way to start. You can easily find the sauce in your local grocery's Asian aisle. This recipe serves one.

Ingredients:

1/4 pound Brussels sprouts

1/2 tablespoon black bean garlic sauce

1/2 tablespoon extra virgin olive oil

Black pepper

Before you start, make sure the Brussels sprouts are cleaned well. Next, trim and cut them lengthwise. Place a skillet over medium high heat and pour oil. Add the sprouts and toss. Let it cook for 3 minutes or until they turn brown.

Next, pour the black bean garlic sauce over the sprouts. Stir until evenly coated. Add black pepper and cook for about 30 seconds more. Serve immediately.

Sesame salmon salad

Packed with salmon flavor with the goodness of sesame, you will surely love this recipe. You can enjoy this salad either warm or cold, it is just as good. It can be served as a light main meal or as lunch. This recipe makes 2 servings.

Ingredients:

1/2 pound wild sockeye salmon fillet

4 won ton wrappers

2 green onions, finely chopped

1 egg

1 small avocado, cut lengthwise

1/2 small head napa cabbage, cut into pieces

1/8 pound trimmed and blanched snow peas

1/2 tablespoon sesame seeds

1/8 cup cilantro, chopped

Vegetable oil

Lemongrass

Chile dressing

Salt

Cut the salmon into half-an-inch thick pieces, and then put in a pot of simmering water with salt. Cover and cook for 5 minutes. Once cooked, drain, take the gray layer underneath it out and set aside to cool.

Put the vegetables into a large pot. Pour oil and place over a medium heat. Set aside once cooked.

Crack the egg into a bowl and add 1 tablespoon of water. Whisk well. Use the egg wash for brushing each side the won tons. Sprinkle with sesame seeds and fry until golden and puffy. Place the cooked won ton on a paper towel then sprinkle with salt.

Place the orange slices, snow peas, cilantro, green onions and cabbage in a large bowl. Pour the dressing and toss. Transfer into serving dishes and place cooked salmon on the side with the avocado slices and fried won ton dishes. Add cilantro leaves to garnish.

Sautéed greens and poached eggs

Ingredients:

> 2 tablespoons of unsalted butter (grass-fed) or ghee

> 2 eggs, poached

> Sea salt

> 2-3 cups of collards, kale, or chard

> 2 tablespoons of sliced almonds or cashews, raw

Cook the greens in a pan containing enough water (an inch). Remove the water and add the ghee or butter. Toss the greens.

Add nuts and salt to taste and put aside. Add the eggs with nuts.

Serve and enjoy.

Taco salad

Ingredients:

The Salad prep:

> A quarter cup of red cabbage, shredded

> Half of an avocado, cut into slices

> A cup of spring lettuce

> A cucumber, sliced

> 2 carrots, shredded

The Taco Mix prep:

> Half of freshly squeezed lime

> A pound of fatty ground beef, organic and grass-fed

> A teaspoon of dried oregano

> A tablespoon of cayenne powder

> 2 tablespoons of unsalted butter, grass-fed or ghee

> Sea salt

The Avocado Dressing prep:

> A quarter cup of apple cider vinegar

> A quarter cup of MCT oil

> A cup of fresh cilantro, chopped

> A quarter cup of fresh lemon juice

> 2 avocados

> 4 cups of cucumber, sliced

> Sea salt

> 4 spring onions

Instructions:

Using a medium-sized pan, cook beef thoroughly and sauté until cooked. Remove the excess fat from the pan and put in the cayenne powder, ghee or butter, oregano, salt, and lime juice. Take it away from the fire and just set it aside.

Combine the ingredients from the salad and put them into plates. Top them off with the beef mix.

Pour the ingredients of the dressing into the blender and mix until creamy and smooth. Drizzle the mixture on top of the salad.

Fish and butternut squash

Ingredients:

Squash preparations:

> A medium-sized butternut squash (seeded and peeled, chopped into 1" cubes)
>
> 4 tablespoons of unsalted butter, grass-fed
>
> 4 medium-sized peeled carrots (chopped into 1" pieces)
>
> Half tablespoon of vinegar, apple cider
>
> A spring onion (chopped into 4 slices)
>
> Sea salt
>
> 2-3 tablespoons of MCT oil

Fish preparations:

> A pound of tilapia filets
>
> 1/4 cup of ground coffee beans
>
> A tablespoon of dried oregano
>
> 1/4 teaspoon of vanilla powder
>
> 3 tablespoons of xylitol
>
> 2 tablespoons of sea salt
>
> A tablespoon of ground turmeric

Heat the oven up 320 degrees F.

Mix the vanilla powder, coffee beans, turmeric, xylitol, salt, and oregano in a container. Pour over fish generously and rub the mixture in.

Put the fish in a dish used for baking (single-layer). Put the dish on the middle rack inside the oven. Bake for about 8-10 minutes or until cooked through.

Steam the carrots and squash until tender. Combine in the blender along with the remaining ingredients, blend to reach the consistency desired.

Stuffed mushrooms

Ingredients:

  4 to 6 big-sized Portobello Mushrooms

  A pound of spicy Italian pork sausage with removed casing

  1.5 pounds of grass-fed, ground beef

  1/2 diced green bell pepper

  3 stalks of celery, diced

  A teaspoon of paprika

  A diced red onion

  Mushroom stems, diced

  2 tablespoons of dried basil

  1/2 teaspoon of cayenne pepper

  Sea salt to taste

  Black pepper

  A tablespoon of tarragon

  1 /4 cup of olive oil

  1 egg (omega-3 enriched)

  6 garlic cloves, crushed 1/4 cup of coconut flour

Preheat the oven up to 400.

With a moist paper towel, carefully wipe off the dirt from the mushrooms, cleaning them under the tap might make them soggy.

Take off the stems and set them aside and carefully scoop out the feathery insides of the mushrooms with a spoon.

Put olive oil on the outsides of the mushrooms and put them in a big glass baking dish, cap down.

Chop up the bell peppers, celery stalks, onions, and mushroom stems.

In a big pot, cook until brown the ground beef and sausage. Add the onions, bell peppers, mushrooms, and celery.

Let it cook until the veggies are tender.

Place the veggie/meat mixture to a blender or food processor and add all the herbs, the coconut flour, egg, and the olive oil.

Blend until the mixture is finely chopped but NOT mushy, it should be chopped fine but still chunky.

Put the mixture into the mushroom caps, filling them completely.

Cook the stuffed mushrooms in the preheated oven until bubbly and brown or around 20 minutes.

Dinner

Your dinner recipes should also provide you with enough protein and a sufficient amount of nutrients. The following is a list of healthy recipes that can help keep you energized and feeling full to avoid hunger pangs and emotional cravings. If you are longing for a light and comforting dinner, you can have a sumptuous soup too.

Chicken and mushrooms

Chicken and mushrooms do not just make a great pair in a creamy soup. They are also a perfect match when it comes to a main dish.

This recipe is good for one. Ingredients:

> 1 boneless chicken breast
>
> 1 cup sliced mushrooms
>
> 1/4 cup chopped green bell pepper
>
> 1 1/2 tablespoon soy sauce
>
> 1/4 tablespoon minced onion
>
> 1/2 teaspoon honey
>
> Garlic powder

Preheat the oven to 350 degrees Fahrenheit. Place the boneless chicken breast on a baking dish. Top with onion flakes.

Mix the soy sauce with the garlic powder in a bowl and pour over the chicken. Cover the baking dish. Place in the pre-heated oven. Let the chicken cook for 30 minutes.

Once cooked, uncover the baking dish and add mushrooms and bell pepper on top. Cover the dish again and place it back inside the oven. Bake until the mushrooms are tender. Take it out and set aside to cool. Serve.

Low carb turkey meatballs

This recipe has an Italian ring to it. Not your usual meatball recipe that uses beef or pork. Rather, this dish's main attraction is turkey! It is only at 166 calories and it is not even that hard to make. This recipe makes 3 meatballs.

Ingredients:

1/2 pound ground turkey

1 egg

1 garlic clove, finely minced

1/8 cup breadcrumbs (made from almond flour)

1/8 cup of chopped onion

1/8 cup chopped parsley

1/4 teaspoon oregano

Salt and pepper

Mix all the ingredients in a large bowl. Divide into three equal portions. Shape each portion into round balls then flatten. Place a non stick pan over medium heat and spray with oil. Cook each side of the meatballs for about 6 minutes or until brown and cooked through. Serve immediately.

Cajun halibut

This is a simple way of cooking halibut steaks. The Cajun flavor mixes well with the fish. It is a sumptuous treat for dinner. This recipe serves two.

Ingredients:

2 halibut steaks

1/8 teaspoon each of ground red pepper, ground black pepper, garlic powder, paprika and salt

Combine the seasonings in a small bowl. Rub both sides of halibut with the seasoning mixture.

Place non-stick skillet over a medium heat. Apply cooking spray then add fish. Cook each side of the halibut for 4 minutes or until cooked through. Serve immediately.

Baked chicken thighs

This is one juicy chicken recipe. And the best part is that it does not call for a heavy prep. This recipe is best served with mixed vegetables and rice, and garnished with chopped fresh parsley. This recipe is good for two.

Ingredients:

    2 chicken thighs

    2 tablespoons soy sauce

    Garlic powder

Arrange the chicken on a baking dish then sprinkle with garlic powder and pour with soy sauce. Place in the oven and cook at 350 degrees Fahrenheit for about an hour.

Beef with broccoli

This stir fry recipe is Chinese inspired. If you want an unusually tasty and delicious dish using simple and easy to find ingredients, this is your best bet. You can enjoy this stir fry with hot brown rice. This recipe is good for one.

Ingredients:

1/4 pound round steak, cut into thick strips

1/4 onion, sliced into wedges

1 cup broccoli florets

1/8 cup water

1 tablespoon cornstarch

1 tablespoon of soy sauce

1 tablespoon vegetable oil

1 tablespoon water, divided

1/4 teaspoon ground ginger

1/8 teaspoon garlic powder

Mix garlic powder with half a tablespoon each of cornstarch and water together in a bowl and add the beef strips. Mix well.

Place a skillet over medium heat and pour half the oil portion. Add coated beef strips and stir fry until tender. Transfer the beef strips on a plate. Then, pour other half portion of oil into the skillet and cook the onion and broccoli. Cook for 4 minutes. Add the beef strips back into the skillet and pour brown sugar, ginger, cornstarch, soy sauce and water. Stir fry for another 2 minutes. Serve immediately.

Sautéed shrimp

This is one tasty dish. It goes well with roasted vegetables. This shrimp recipe serves two.

Ingredients:

1/2 pound shrimp, peeled and deveined

1 tablespoon freshly squeezed lemon juice

1 tablespoon chopped parsley

1 teaspoon of olive oil

1/2 teaspoon herb seasoning

Salt and pepper

Place skillet over a medium heat and pour oil. Stir in shrimp and saute for 1 minute. Sprinkle with salt, herb seasoning and pepper. Drizzle with lemon juice and keep stirring. Cook for 4 minutes more. Sprinkle chopped parsley before transferring to a serving dish.

Lemony chicken soup

A yummy soup that can provide comfort especially in cold weather, this is a perfect way to end a long week. You can make it so the soup forms drops by not stirring the eggs. But if you want something different from an egg drop soup, stir in the egg so it does not form. This recipe makes 3 to 4 servings.

Ingredients:

1 cup of cooked chicken, cut into half inch thick pieces

1 cup chicken broth

1 egg

1 chicken bouillon cube

1 sliced carrot

1/2 small onion, minced

1 tablespoon freshly squeezed lemon juice

Oregano

Salt and pepper

Place the chicken broth, chicken bouillon cube and 1 cup water into a Dutch oven. Let it boil the chicken. Simmer for 20 minutes. Pour in lemon juice along with the egg. Sprinkle with salt, pepper and oregano. Serve while hot.

Chicken pot pie

Ingredients:

Filling preparations:

> 3 slices of diced bacon
>
> A diced carrot
>
> A chopped onion
>
> A clove of crushed garlic
>
> A diced stalk of celery
>
> A 14-ounce can of coconut milk
>
> 1/4 cup of cut green beans
>
> A cup of chicken stock
>
> A teaspoon of salt
>
> 2 tablespoons of arrowroot
>
> A tablespoon of poultry seasoning
>
> 1/2 teaspoon of pepper
>
> 2 cups of chopped cooked chicken

Use a pot to cook the bacon until crispy.

Put in the carrot, onion, garlic, and celery, and cook it for 5 minutes. Make sure to scrape the bottom of the pan.

Add the coconut milk, chicken stock, poultry seasoning, pepper green beans salt, and chicken and bring to a boil.

Simmer and add in the arrowroot 1 tablespoon at a time until mixed.

Continue simmering until the mixture is thick.

Pour into an 8-by-12 inch baking dish.

Dough preparations:

Ingredients:

> A cup of tapioca flour

1/4 teaspoon of baking soda

1/4 cup of coconut flour

3 tablespoon of butter or coconut oil

Half teaspoon of cream of tartar

Half cup of water, boiling

Half teaspoon of salt

Strain all of the dry ingredients. Mix in butter to the dry ingredients and mix them to make crumbles. Pour in the hot water.

Fashion into a ball and press it into a flat rectangle.

Place over pot pie ingredients and bake at 400 for 10 minutes.

Beef Burgundy

Ingredients:

>3 lbs. of beef cut into cubes for about 2 inches each
>
>1/4 lb. of bacon
>
>4tbsps. of butter
>
>1/4 tsp. of pepper
>
>1 and a half tsps. of salt
>
>2 sliced carrots
>
>2 tbsps. of almond flour
>
>A tbsp. of tomato paste
>
>A sliced onion
>
>A tablespoon fresh thyme or dried
>
>2 cloves garlic, finely chopped
>
>3 cups full-bodied red wine
>
>A tbsp. of fresh parsley, finely chopped
>
>A bay leaf
>
>A lb. of white or brown crimini mushrooms
>
>2 1/2 cups beef stock

Preheat your oven to 425.

Prepare the bacon by cutting them into short strips. Sauté the bacon in a deep saucepan with a tablespoon of butter. Cook until the bacon is cooked, making sure it is not crispy.

Use a paper towel to pat dry the beef. Add the beef into the bacon in 3 to 4 batches. Make sure to cook until each batch of meat is brown before removing from pan.

Put the meat and bacon aside in a casserole baking dish. You will be using this in the oven later on. Add the pepper, salt, and almond flour over the meat in an even manner.

Cook the meat by baking it in the oven for 10 minutes and do not put a cover on it. In this way, the flour is absorbed into the meat and might make a slight crust.

Take it from the oven and lower the heat to 325.

Mix a tablespoon of butter to the remaining fat from the bacon and meat in the saucepan. Sauté the onion and carrots for 8 minutes or until soft.

Add the garlic, tomato paste, bay leaf, thyme, and parsley.

Mix in the beef broth and wine. Bring this to a boil and let it simmer for about 3 to 5 minutes. Put the meat on a casserole pan and pour in the mixture.

Put the lid on the dish. Bake in the oven for about 2 and a half hours. The meat should be done if you can pull it apart with a fork.

Sautee the mushrooms and remaining butter in a pan while the meat is cooking.

Once the meat is cooked, take the casserole pan from the oven.

Drain the liquid from the pan by using a colander.

Bring the liquid to a boil and simmer for 8 to 10 minutes. Pour over meat and mushrooms. Garnish with parsley and serve.

The Shepherd's Pie

Ingredients:

The Filling prep:

> Half cup of frozen peas
>
> A tablespoon of dried parsley
>
> A pound of ground beef or lamb (grass-fed), can also be a combination of the two
>
> A teaspoon of dried rosemary
>
> A medium-sized onion
>
> A clove of garlic
>
> 1 and 1/2 tablespoons of tomato paste
>
> 2 carrots
>
> 2 tablespoons of butter (grass-fed), beef tallow (grass-fed), or hog lard (pastured)
>
> 2 celery stalks
>
> Sea salt
>
> Salt and pepper

The Mashed Topping prep:

> Your choice of: 1 and 1/2 pounds of potatoes, 1 and 1/2 pounds of root vegetables of your choice (must be mashable), A head of cauliflower, or 1 and 1/2 pounds of sweet potatoes
>
> 1/4 cup of coconut milk (full-fat) or heavy cream
>
> A tablespoon of ghee or grass-fed butter
>
> Salt and pepper to taste

Using a saucepan, boil the chopped cauliflower, potatoes, or your root vegetables. Once done, drain the water and add the remaining ingredients of the mashed topping prep and start mashing.

Preheat your oven up to 350 degrees.

Clean and chop the onion, garlic, celery, and carrots. In a heavy pan, sauté the tallow, lard, or butter adding a pinch of salt. Once cooked, put the tomato paste, peas, and other spices.

Make a space in the middle of the heavy pan. Cook the ground lamb or beef adding salt. Break them up to pieces.

Put the mixture into separate oven-safe plates or containers and add mashed potatoes and/or veggies on top. Cook by baking for 20 to 30 minutes.

Conclusion

I hope that you have learned all the secrets of the ketogenic diet - the principles behind it, how it is beneficial to weight loss, the best recipes as well as the best practices to adopt to make your attempt to lose weight and burn more body fats successful.

Your next step is to apply everything that you have learned from this book in your daily life. No matter how hectic your lifestyle it, take time to make use of the recipes presented in this book to continually practice ketogenic diet.

Forget about starvation since ketogenic diet allows you to eat satisfyingly. Burn fats, lose weight fast by starting your new lifestyle today.

Good luck!

Bonus Recipes

TABLE OF CONTENTS

Chocolate pudding

Ingredients:

> 4 tbsps. of hardwood xylitol or stevia
>
> 4 cups of divided coconut milk that is BpA-free
>
> 2 tsps. of vanilla powder
>
> A tbsp. of gelatin, grass-fed
>
> A tbsp of MCT oil
>
> 3/4 cup of chocolate powder
>
> 1/4 cup of macadamia nuts
>
> 4 tbsps. of butter, unsalted

Instructions:

Heat a cup of the coconut milk, the stevia, and the gelatin in the pan. Do this over heat of medium-grade until all have dissolved.

Put the remaining three cups of coconut milk in a food processor or blender with the chocolate powder, vanilla, oil, and butter then blend.

Add the mixture of coconut milk and gelatin to your blender. Blend until combined, adding macadamia nuts is optional.

Put the blender contents into ramekins or muffin tins and store in the refrigerator for 1 hour.

Top it with nuts (optional).

Fudge

Ingredients:

Half cup of coconut oil

Half cup of smooth almond butter

Half cup of cocoa powder (high quality)

Half teaspoon of vanilla

Half cup of maple syrup/raw honey

Melt the coconut oil in the microwave or overheat.

Mix all ingredients in a blender or food processor.

Pour the contents into silicon muffin cups or muffin cups lined with paper. Make sure to fill half of an inch to make about 10 servings.

Store in the fridge for half an hour. You can also put it in the freezer for about 10 minutes.

Remove from the fridge once firm and put in an airtight container and put them back in the fridge for storage.

Lemon balls

Ingredients:

Zest of 1 big lemon

A cup of desiccated coconut

A cup of cashews, raw

Sea salt

Half tsp. of natural vanilla extract, concentrated

Extra serving of desiccated coconut

2 tbsp. of maple syrup

Mix all the ingredients in a blender or a food processor. Put in the cashews first, the desiccated coconut, the lemon zest, vanilla extract, salt, and finally, the maple syrup. You can add more desiccated coconut if desired.

Shape the mixture into balls and store in the fridge to freeze a little bit.

Serve cold.

Creamy coconut ice cream

Ingredients:

2 teaspoon of vanilla

3 tablespoon + 2 teaspoon/50 g MCT oil

4 yolks aside from the whole eggs

4 pastured whole eggs

A tablespoon/80-160 g of erythritol or xylitol

1 gram of vitamin C/ascorbic acid (you can also use lime juice or apple cider vinegar, 10 drops)

Half cup/100g of water or ice

7 tablespoons/100g of coconut oil

7 tablespoons/100g of butter, grass-fed

1/4 to half cup of chocolate powder (low-toxin), optional

Mix all ingredients in the blender except the water or ice. You need to make sure the mixture reaches a creamy texture before adding in the water.

Pour in water or the ice and continue blending until fully incorporated. The ideal consistency is of that of a yogurt or ice cream.

Put the mix into the ice cream maker. Turn on the ice cream maker.

Coconut pudding with chia

Chia is a reliable ingredient for low carb recipes on the go. The gelatinous texture of the chia combined with the softness of blueberry is a match made in heaven. This recipe is good for one.

For the ingredients, you need the following:

> 2 tablespoons chia seed
>
> 2 tablespoons unsweet coconut
>
> 1/2 cup water
>
> 1/2 teaspoon vanilla

Put the chia seeds, coconut, water and vanilla in the blender. Process the ingredients until smooth. Pour the mixture into a bowl. Let it cool in the fridge for 15 to 30 minutes or until you have a thick mixture. Take it out.

For additional flavor, you can also sprinkle the pudding with nuts.

The Ketogenic Cacao

Ingredients:

Half cup of coconut milk, full-fat

Half cup of water

2 tablespoons of unsalted butter

1/4 teaspoon of vanilla extract

2 tablespoons of regular or raw cacao powder

Cinnamon

2 teaspoon of raw honey, if wanted

Mix the coconut milk and water and bring to a boil in a saucepan.

Combine the boiling mix with the other ingredients and put them in a mixing bowl.

Mix in a blender or hand mixer, wait until frothy.

Pour into a mug and serve.

Chocolate avocado mousse

Ingredients:

    2 small very ripe avocados

    1/4 cup water

    3 tablespoons cocoa (9 grams)

    6 tablespoons granular Splenda or equivalent liquid Splenda

    1/2 teaspoon vanilla

    Pinch salt

In a food processor, process ingredients for 4-5 minutes. Chill.

Coconut macaroons

Ingredients:

> 4 large egg whites
>
> 1 tsp. vanilla
>
> 1/4 tsp. cream of tartar
>
> 1/8 tsp. salt
>
> 1 cup erythritol
>
> 16 ounces finely shredded, unsweetened dried coconut
>
> 8 ounces cream cheese, softened
>
> 2 ounces heavy cream
>
> 2 ounces sugar free white chocolate syrup
>
> 2 ounces mini chocolate chips

Preheat oven to 325 degrees.

Line 2 large baking sheets with parchment paper.

In a large mixing bowl, on low, beat together egg whites, vanilla, cream of tartar and salt until soft peaks form.

Add erythritol a tablespoon at a time. Beat until stiff peaks form.

Fold in coconut.

Beat together cream cheese and cream until smooth.

Mix in syrup.

Add in coconut mixture, a little at a time.

Fold in chocolate chips.

Using a small ice cream scoop, place mixture on baking sheet.

Bake 20-25 minutes. Turn off oven leaving cookies in for 30 minutes.

Move to wire rack.

Let cool.

Raspberry coconut pancakes

Ingredients:

Pancakes:

> 2 large eggs
>
> 1 tbsp. fine coconut flour
>
> 2 tbsp. desiccated coconut (unsweetened)
>
> 1/4 tsp. baking soda
>
> 3 tbsp. coconut milk
>
> 1/2 tsp. pure vanilla bean extract
>
> 1 tbsp. extra virgin coconut oil
>
> 3-6 drops liquid Stevia extract

Topping:

> 1/2 cup plain organic yogurt
>
> 1/2 tsp. pure vanilla bean extract
>
> 1/3 cup fresh raspberries
>
> 1 tsp. desiccated coconut (unsweetened)

Beat eggs.

In a separate bowl, combine coconut flour, coconut, vanilla bean extract and baking soda.

Add to eggs.

Add coconut a little at a time.

Mix well.

Add sweetener.

In a separate bowl, mix the yogurt.

Grease a pan with coconut oil and turn heat to low. Pour half a ladle of batter into the pan. Flip when bubbles form.

Cook for 1 minute.

Top with coconut.

Peanutty frozen dessert

Ingredients:

      1 cup cottage cheese

      1 scoop protein powder

      2 Tbsp. peanut butter

      2 Tbsp. heavy cream

      6 drops Splenda

In a food processor, blend together ingredients except protein powder.

When smooth mix in protein powder, blend to remove chunks.

Freeze for 40 minutes.